# Stress

*A Natural Solution to Completely Manage and Cure your Stress and Negative Thoughts for Good!*

**Robert S. Lee**

© **Copyright 2019 by Robert S. Lee- All rights reserved.**

This document is geared toward providing exact and reliable information in regard to the topic and issue covered. The publication is sold with the idea that the publisher is not required to render accounting, officially permitted, or otherwise, qualified services. If advice is necessary, legal or professional, a practiced individual in the profession should be ordered.

- From a Declaration of Principles which was accepted and approved equally by a Committee of the American Bar Association and a Committee of Publishers and Associations.

In no way is it legal to reproduce, duplicate, or transmit any part of this document in either electronic means or in printed format. Recording of this publication is strictly prohibited and any storage of this document is not allowed unless with written permission from the publisher. All rights reserved.

The information provided herein is stated to be truthful and consistent, in that any liability, in terms of inattention or otherwise, by any usage or abuse of any policies, processes, or directions contained within is the solitary and utter responsibility of the recipient reader. Under no circumstances will any legal responsibility or blame be held against the publisher for any reparation, damages, or monetary loss due to the information herein, either directly or indirectly.

Respective authors own all copyrights not held by the publisher.

The information herein is offered for informational purposes solely, and is universal as so. The presentation of the information is without contract or any type of guarantee assurance.

The trademarks that are used are without any consent, and the publication of the trademark is without permission or backing by the trademark owner. All trademarks and brands within this book are for clarifying purposes only and are the owned by the owners themselves, not affiliated with this document.

## Contents

Chapter 1. The Importance of Stress Relief.......1

Chapter 2. Coping Techniques for Stress ......... 5

Chapter 3. Using Meditation to Help Out .......16

Chapter 4. Basic Herbal Teas to Make............ 25

Chapter 5. Herbal Baths & Why They Work .. 36

Chapter 6. Essential Oils for Anxiety & Stress. ............................................................................ 44

Chapter 7. Natural Habits You Can Stack ...... 55

Chapter 8. Stress Relieving Face Masks.......... 65

Chapter 9. Extra Tips & Tricks to Help .......... 76

# Chapter 1. The Importance of Stress Relief

Stress management, also known as stress relief, is extremely important to your health. You need to reduce the stress in your everyday life to live a healthier life as a happier you. If you're too stressed, you're going to lower your immune system and open yourself up to a large range of illnesses and ailments, and that is anything from a common cold to heart disease. You can't be a healthy you without your stress being in check.

**What Stress Does:**

You put yourself at risk with stress, and most people don't even think about the stress in their life until they're close to a burn out, which could resort in horrible consequences to your health and mental stability. Your brain deals with a physical and chemical change that affects its functioning when you're stressed. Chemicals in your brain will start to rise, and you'll turn into a fight or flight situation, where adrenaline is released. It can increase your blood pressure, weaken your immune system, and even increase your heart rate. It can cause ulcers, asthma, heart disease, stroke and many other health related issues if you undergo stress or hold onto it too long.

It increases your chances of heart attack, and you may attempt to adapt to the stress that is ongoing in your life, but without the proper coping methods and stress reduction methods, then you'll find it doesn't actually work. You may build a mental tolerance for some of the stress, but you still deal with physical reactions that are commonly ignored. This includes the tensing of your muscles, headaches or migraines, and even indigestion. Of course, it will also physically affect which nutrients your intestines get to absorb. This can cause you to eat more or less than you normally do, which can cause heartburn, acid reflux, vomiting, pain, nausea and even diarrhea.

You even experience psychological effects from stress, and it can lead to both emotional and mental disorders. This includes many phobias, panic attacks, anxiety, and it can even lead to depression. This can disrupt your decision making, focus, and ability to remember things, even important things because your overall memory suffers. It can even cause you to be more moody and irritable with a quick temper. This can cause you to have conflicts in your relationship, be too quick to anger, and feel insecure about various things.

**You Can Manage It:**

Stress isn't something you just have to put up with. You can deal with it in a healthy manner, and there are many coping mechanisms, herbs, and habits that you can put together to make sure that you're dealing with your stress instead of just putting up with it and bottling it up. From making sure you get adequate sleep to using essential oils to help you relieve stress, there are many routes you can take to make sure stress isn't a problem that really troubles you. Stress management will help to make sure that you have everything you need to be a healthier, happier person, and it can reduce your chances of ailments and diseases and even help you to age gracefully.

# Chapter 2. Coping Techniques for Stress

Stress hits you no matter what life you live, and it's something that's sadly unavoidable. You'll find that you need to stay focused and motivated if you want to have a complete and fulfilling life. You need to ditch the unhealthy coping methods, such as turning to drugs, alcohol, or even just food. You shouldn't take out your stress on another because healthy coping methods are easy to use, and this chapter helps to make sure you have all the tools you need to do so.

**Coping Technique #1 Perform Deep Breathing**

This is a simple coping mechanism that you can do anywhere at any time. You don't have to wait until you get home, and you don't even need a quiet place to do it in. if you're in a place that's too noisy to concentrate, remember to just count your breathing. The best method is to count up to ten, and if you have the time and your stress is really pressing in on you, then you'll want to count back down to zero as well. Keep your eyes closed if possible, and this will help you to center your internal self, helping to block out the stressors of the external world.

**Coping Technique #2 Go for a Jog**

This may seem counterproductive, but if you have the time and you're stressed out, go for a jog. When you're stressed, it's likely that you'll become angry, antsy, or just that your adrenaline will spike. It's important to get it out in a healthy manner, which will help to lower your temper, bring you back into balance with your mental self, and burn off the energy in a productive way.

Jogging or running is a great way to do so, but going for a walk will help as well. It usually helps you to remove yourself from the problem directly as well, giving you time to reflect and calm down so that you can handle the situation in a healthy manner with a clear mind.

**Coping Technique #3 Listen to Music**

If you don't like music, then this isn't for you. However, there are many different types of music that you can listen to. It doesn't have to be something soft or soothing, either. It should always be music that you enjoy. Just take a moment to listen to a song or two, and then you'll find that if its music you truly like, and it's not depressing or angry, then it'll actually help to relieve some of your stress and clear your mind so that you can think properly. You'll still have to make sure that you face your stressors head on later, but stepping back from the stress for a moment helps.

## Coping Technique #4 Make the List of Good

If you have a pencil and paper or even your phone, then you'll want to physically write it down, but making a list will actually help you. Just make a list of the good things that's happened that day, no matter how small they are. You can put it from getting a discount on something you wanted to buy to getting a call from someone you love. There is usually at least one good thing, usually many more, that have happened to you in a day before the stress builds up, and it's important to recognize them if you want to lessen the effects of stress in your life.

## Coping Technique #5 Take 30 Minutes for Yourself

If you have the time and you're too stressed out, try to actually find thirty minutes for yourself. You don't need to try and take it just then if you really can't. Of course, it's usually better if you make sure that you have a half hour to do what you want every day. This may mean that you need to say no to people and take time just to yourself, but it's what you need to make sure that your stress is managed. It'll help you to have a more positive outlook so that you can cope with your stress in a healthy manner.

## Coping Technique #6 Find Something to Laugh At

This can be hard to do if you're too stressed, but whenever you can, you need to find something to laugh at if you're extremely stressed. It can be a picture on your phone, a joke you heard earlier, or just the irony of your situation. Laughter really is a great way to release the stress and tension from your body. It can also help to make sure that you aren't feeling too depressed with your life, and this can help to keep chronic stress or depression at bay. It can even help to stave of panic attacks or anxiety attacks.

## Coping Technique #7 Recognize Living in the Now

Many people don't live in the now. Often, you're too consumed with your worries of the past or the future, and you can't really see the present for what it really is. You can't see the good in the now if all you're thinking about is what has come and what is to come. You need to realize that there is beauty in the present.

Take a moment to find the beauty in your surroundings, recognize your thoughts, and recognize who you're with and why. This is living in the now, and it'll help you to feel more centered and less pressure from the stressors in your life.

## Coping Technique #8 Write It All Down

Write everything down that is starting to annoy you, stress you, or even depress you. Of course, you'll find that writing it down isn't always possible in the moment. However, you should try to write down what's bothering you at least once daily. It doesn't have to be a list of your bad experiences that day, but it can be as simple as a journal entry.

It'll help to put your life into perspective, and sometimes perspective changes everything. You're less stressed if your stressor doesn't seem as big or as important. When you write it down, it's more likely you'll come up with a solution to your problems as well, since the feelings aren't there, but the actual problem is in black and white.

## Coping Technique #9 Use a Positive Affirmation

Positive affirmations are easy to use, but they're sometimes hard to figure out which one is best for you. Try to tell yourself an affirmation based on what you're feeling. If your stress is making you feel insecure, then say something that will help to chase those insecurities away. It can be something as simple as telling yourself that you're confident, beautiful, or that you're living in the now.

Make an affirmation based now hat you need, and repeat it to yourself. If you have a mirror available, it usually works best to repeat it out loud in front of the mirror. Try to say it out loud at least, but saying it quietly to yourself works as well. This will keep stress from keeping you down or ruining your day, which will make it smaller and easier to handle overall.

## Coping Technique #10 Account for Your Feelings

You always need to account for your feelings. There are many reasons that you're feeling stressed, and even if some emotions are irrational, it'll only get worse if you're trying to suppress them. Suppressing your feelings will actually add to stress, which will make everything worse. It'll make you feel like things are weighing you down, and so you need to recognize your feelings.

Try to recognize that you're feeling an emotion, and then try to ask yourself why. This will help you to process those feelings healthily, and it'll then help to make sure no more stress stems from the emotion or even that the stress that caused it is solved, depending on the situation.

# Chapter 3. Using Meditation to Help Out

If you know meditation, then you probably already know that it can help with stress, and it can help anywhere you are. There are some meditation techniques that you'll have to use while you're at home, so you'll need to set time aside for them. There are many benefits of meditation, and stress reduction is one of them. It will help your mental, emotional and overall health, including your physical. It'll give you a sense of inner peace, which is what stress takes away.

**Affecting the Emotional & Mental Symptoms of Stress:**

Meditation allows you to clear away the information that's building up and overloading your system, which happen every day and contributes to the majority of your stress. It'll help you to look at everything in a new way with a new perspective when you meditate, including the stressful situations that you're experiencing.

It will help you build skills that help you to manage your stress, increase your self-awareness, and reduce your negative emotions. It also helps you to stay in the present, and it keeps you from dwelling on the past or the future, which helps to reduce stress overall.

**Affecting Physical Symptoms of Stress:**

Meditation can help you to affect your physical self as well. It can help not only to stave off depression but also high blood pressure, chronic pain, sleep problems and disorders, anxiety and anxiety disorders, and even heart disease and asthma. There are many pros and cons of meditation, but the pros usually far outweigh the cons, which usually include the time that meditation takes.

However, if you are not meditation properly you may worsen the symptoms that that are associated with physical conditions. It may cause your high blood pressure to spike if you are not meditating properly because of instead of observing something that is bothering you, you may dwell on it, which will increase your heart rate and adrenaline. When done right, it'll calm both of those things.

**Meditation #1 Breathing Building Blocks**

Breathing is important, and it keeps you alive, but meditation isn't simply about breathing even when it includes breathing exercises. Breathing exercises are done because they are the building blocks of meditation. You need to learn to breathe properly. This doesn't mean that you need to breathe too deeply or too shallowly. Instead, you'll find that you need to breathe normally but with a concentration on your breathing to use breathing as a meditation exercise, especially when dealing with your stress.

Start by sitting in a quiet place in comfortable clothes, and make sure that you're sitting in a position that is comfortable as well. You can even meditate laying down if you feel like that is most beneficial. Start by taking a deep breath, centering yourself. Make sure to concentrate on the feeling of breathing. Concentrate on how it expands your lungs and how it travels from your nose, to your lungs, and back out through your mouth. If you are having a hard time concentrating, you may find its best to just count your breathing, which will help to center your focus where it needs to be.

Don't let stray thoughts be more than acknowledged. You don't want to interact with your thoughts or you will only increase your stress. Then, you can make sure that you breathe in and out while dismissing what is stressing you. This works great if you are in a stressful situation, and if you can't sit down to meditate, doing so with closed eyes in a quiet area, such as your work space or your car, will work just as well.

**Meditation #2 Mantra Meditation**

Mantra meditation is also commonly used when you are in a stressful situation or trying to deal with stress on a certain level or about a certain thing. Mantra meditation is where you silently repeat a mantra to yourself during a meditational like state which you enter into. A mantra can be a calming word, phrase, or even just a thought that will help you to implement positive thoughts or feelings while keeping distracting thoughts at bay. Make sure to find a mantra that works for you. It can be a phrase that you're telling yourself, just like a positive affirmation.

You can tell yourself that you're brave, you're strong, and you'll get through it. It can be a simple word like confidence, bravery, or anything else that really speaks to you. You can take a moment to just close your eyes and center yourself, or you can use it can be when you put your time aside at the beginning, end, or even during the day that will help you to make sure that you are using mantra meditation to help with your stress to its fullest.

## Meditation #3 Meditation of Emotions

This is commonly a mindful meditation, and it's usually where you're being mindful of your emotions. This is where you recognize the emotions you're feeling, which are commonly contributing to stress. However, this is not a meditation you should try to do when you're busy. It's often too difficult to properly perform with something that is distracting around you. It's usually best if you have the time to sit down so that you can properly sort out your emotions. If you are interrupted, it could only cause more stress, which will add onto the issue without actually helping you.

To start meditation of emotions, also known as mindfulness meditation of emotions, then you're going to want to get in a quiet place with comfortable clothes and in a comfortable position. Then, you're going to want to center yourself. This can usually be done with meditation breathing exercises, which is why it's considered the building block to many meditation practices. Once you feel you're centered, instead of dismissing the thoughts that come by, which are usually the ones that are bugging you, you're going to want to acknowledge them and let yourself feel the emotion from the thought or memory that is bothering you.

Acknowledge that the emotion is present, and ask yourself why. Ask yourself how the emotion makes you feel. Replay the memory of what caused the emotion without dwelling on it. Tell yourself that it's okay to feel that way, but remind yourself that it's fixable. That this problem doesn't have to lead to a negative emotion. This will help to remove the stress that the emotion is causing you, and it can bring about a new perspective on the stressful situation.

**Just Remember:**

Meditation takes time. It doesn't have to be a full half hour in each sitting, but it's important to make the time in your life to help make sure that you have the time you need to help make sure you are meditating properly. It's good to set aside at least ten or fifteen minutes a day, and you can do this twice a day. However, longer meditation sessions have been known to help more than shorter ones because it gives you the needed time to process what you are feeling and process your stress in a healthy manner. This is why meditation is another coping mechanism that can help with stress, but only if it's done properly.

# Chapter 4. Basic Herbal Teas to Make

Herbs are great at making sure that you have something you can take that's natural that will physically help you to cope with stress and the affects that stress has on your body. Of course, one of the best ways to make sure to take these herbs is through a tea. It doesn't have to be warm, but warm tea has been proven to help more.

However, you can ice your tea if you are taking them a little more often. In that case, just make the tea in advance, making sure to dissolve the honey into it, and put it in the refrigerator or freezer to chill. You should always use natural or raw honey as no sugar has been added, and sugar affects your body negatively. Too much sugar consumption can actually cause your body to go out of balance, contributing to stress instead of helping it.

## Tea #1 Lemon Balm Green Tea

Lemon balm is also a culinary herb, but it's medicinal as well. It's actually from the mint family, and it has lemony and minty scent that lends to its name. It was commonly used by both the Romans and the Greeks, and it's known to reduce your anxiety and lower your stress levels. A lemon balm tea, especially when paired with green tea which is known to have a crisp taste, will help you to reduce the stress that you're experiencing.

Ingredients:

1. 1 Tablespoon Green Tea Leaves
2. 2 Teaspoons Lemon Balm, Dried
3. 1 ½ Teaspoon Honey, Raw

*Directions:*

1. Boil a single cup of water, adding in your lemon balm and green tea, and then reduce to a simmer. Let it simmer for five to seven minutes, turning off the heat and straining.
2. After straining, add in your honey and mix well. Drink while hot, and add more honey if needed.

**Tea #2 Passionflower Tea**

Passionflower is actually know to be a sedative, so once again, you may want to add green tea or white tea in it. You will also want to pair it with a fruit, which orange zest is used in this recipe, to give it a wonderful taste. It's supposed to help reduce anxiety, stress, and promote healthy sleep. This can help if your stress is causing you to lose sleep or not sleep peacefully.

Ingredients:

1. 1 ½ Teaspoons Passionflower, Dried
2. 3-4 Mint Leaves, Fresh
3. 1 ½ Teaspoons Honey, Raw
4. ½ Teaspoon Orange Zest

*Directions:*

1. Take a cup of water, boiling it and adding passionflower, mint leaves, and your orange zest. Let simmer for four to six minutes after reducing to a simmer. Next, strain out all of your herbs.
2. Add in honey and stir until dissolved as warm. Add lemon if desired.

**Tea #3 Holy Basil**

You'll often find basil right in your kitchen cabinet. Use some holy basil to help with your stress levels as well, and it's great in tea form. However, once again orange zest is added because it adds flavor while being easy to get ahold of. Many people will dry and grate orange peel just to make their own. It's a simple tea to make, and it's known to help stave off depression, lighten your mood, and manage your stress.

Ingredients:

1. 2 Tablespoons Holy Basil, Dried
2. 1 Teaspoon Orange Zest
3. 2 Teaspoon Honey, Raw

*Directions:*

1. Start by boiling your cup of water before throwing in your bail and orange zest. Let simmer for four to six minutes.

2. Strain out all herbs, and then add in your honey. Drink warm or let cool.

**Tea #4 Chamomile Tea**

This is a simple tea, and often you can get it premade to help make sure that you can use it more often by making it a little simpler. However, chamomile is a mild sedative, so it can cause many people to get sleepy. It's a nighttime tea that is great for stress relief, and it'll help with the effects of anxiety and stress both mentally and physically.

Ingredients:

1. 2 Tablespoons Chamomile Flowers, Dried
2. 1 Teaspoon Honey, Raw

*Directions:*

1. Some people will add mint, but all you need to do is boil a cup of water, adding in your chamomile before reducing it to simmer for four to six minutes.
2. Strain the chamomile out, and then add honey and lemon juice if desired.

## Tea #5 Lavender & Chamomile Stress Relief

Most people don't like a tea made of lavender on its own, but it'll help as well. Many people prefer the taste of a chamomile and lavender mix, making it yet another nighttime tea to help you with stress. Lavender is a wild flower, but it's also an herb that is known to relieve stress and tension in your body, which will help with both the stress itself and the effects on your physical self.

Ingredients:

1. 1 Tablespoon Chamomile Flowers, Dried
2. 2 Teaspoons Lavender Flowers, Dried
3. 1 ½ Teaspoons Honey, Raw

*Directions:*

1. Boil your water, which should only be a cup, adding in the chamomile and lavender flowers as you reduce it to a simmer. Let simmer for five to seven minutes, and then strain.
2. Add in honey, and add lemon juice if desired before drinking. It mixes better when warm, but you can drink warm or chilled.

**Tea #6 Green Tea & Lavender**

Lavender and green tea make a great combination, and you can even add a dash of lemon or mint if you need to. Green tea is a mild stimulant, just like lavender can sometimes act like a mild sedative, so they often balance each other out. Of course, you'll find that green tea is known to relieve anxiety just as well.

Ingredients:

1. 2 Teaspoons Green Tea Leaves
2. 2 Teaspoons Lavender Flowers, Dried
3. 1 Teaspoon Honey, Raw

*Directions:*

1. Boil your one cup of water, adding in your tea leaves and lavender flowers. Reduce to a simmer and simmer for five to seven minutes.
2. Strain out your herbs, and add in your honey to taste.

## Tea #7 Green Tea & Licorice Root

Licorice root is a great way to reduce your stress and anxiety, and it provides a unique and crisp taste when you add it to green tea. Of course, you'll find that many people prefer to add a little dash of cinnamon for flavor. Licorice root helps to handle your stress by giving you a natural hormone, which is an alternative to cortisone, and it helps you to handle stressful situation. It will even help to normalize your blood sugar and adrenal gland. It is meant to sooth the mind, and is best taken when you are drinking your tea hot.

Ingredients:

1. 1 Teaspoon Licorice Root, Dried
2. 2 Teaspoons Green Tea Leaves
3. 3-4 Mint Leaves, Fresh
4. 1 ½ Teaspoons Honey, Raw

*Directions:*

1. Boil your cup of water, and add in your green tea, mint, and licorice root. Reduce and let simmer for five to six minutes.
2. Strain, and add in honey and cinnamon if desired.

# Chapter 5. Herbal Baths & Why They Work

Bathing can actually be more than just for cleaning, and it's great if you are trying to reduce your stress if you're using an herbal bath. If you're trying to keep them from sticking to your skin, it's best to put them in a sachet. However, it can be applied directly to the water. The aroma of an herbal bath is what's meant to relax and sooth you. Try not to use extremely hot water, as this can be drying to your skin, but you are going to want warm water so that you feel better. There are some herbal baths that are okay to use during the day, but remember that most are best at night, since it'll help you to sleep, and a hot bath promotes better sleep to begin with.

## Herbal Bath #1 An Earthy Herbal Blend

Rosemary and sage are a great way to help make sure that you're getting an earthy scent that's still going to help you with your stress. They're also two herbs that you can get commonly, and many people already have them in their kitchen. Just throw them into the bath with you, and you'll find that even dried herbs work, but fresh is usually better. Rosemary will also help to make sure that your aches and pains are melting away along with your stress, and the sage helps to release built up emotions that are caused by stress.

Ingredients:

1. 5 Tablespoons Sage, Dried
2. 4 Tablespoons Rosemary, Dried
3. 5-7 Drops Cedarwood Essential Oil

*Directions:*

1. Just mix it into warm water, and soak for twenty to thirty minutes.

**Herbal Bath #2 Simple Chamomile**

Chamomile is top on the list to help you sleep and relax your body and mind, helping stress to just dissolve away in the water. With warm water, it's like soaking in chamomile tea, and you're sure to get all the relief you need. It's simple to make, and it's all you need. Of course, chamomile flowers usually work best, but you can add chamomile essential oil for an added boost as well if desired.

Ingredients:

1. ¼ Cup Chamomile Flowers
2. 3-5 Drops Chamomile Essential Oil

*Directions:*

1. Run warm to hot water, depending upon preference, and pour in the flowers, soaking for twenty to thirty minutes.

**Herbal Bath #3 Basil & Jasmine**

If you're looking for a bath that doesn't have to be used at bed time, then this would be the herbal bath for you. Basil acts as a mild stimulant, and it'll help you to feel relaxed and yet refreshed and ready to conquer whatever you need to. Jasmine is more of a heady scent, and it'll work on your muscles as well as your mind. Having the flowers bruised will release more of their properties, helping you to relax even more.

Ingredients:

1. ¼ Cup Jasmine Flowers, Bruised
2. 4 Tablespoons Basil, Dried or Fresh

*Directions:*

1. Run the hot water, and then just add in the flowers and basil.

## Herbal Bath #4 Lavender Bath

A lavender bath is relaxing, and the smell of lavender can help you with tension, headaches, migraines, anxiety, depression and even stress. Many people will add an essential oil of their choice, but dried or fresh lavender flowers are great if you're looking for an herbal bath to help you relax for the night and make sure that your stress won't bother you or interrupt your sleep.

Ingredients:

1. ¼ Cup Lavender Flowers, Dried

*Directions:*

1. Run a hot bath, adding in the lavender flowers. Remember that if you decide to use fresh flowers, pack them down and make sure they're bruised before adding them to the water.

## Herbal Bath #5 Lemon Balm & Mint

Mint is refreshing, and it'll help you to be awake and ready to go. However, lemon balm is soothing, and it's known to help with depression, anxiety or even stress. Adding it to your bath is just as helpful as adding it to a tea, and it's easy to make. Having fresh leaves is always best.

Ingredients:

1. 15-20 Mint Leaves, Fresh
2. ¼ Cup Lemon Balm, Fresh

*Directions:*

1. Draw your hot bath, and add in the herbs, letting yourself soak for twenty to thirty minutes. Try to leave your troubles behind, but these herbs are sure to make that a little easier.

## Herbal Bath #6 Rose & Lavender

Lavender flowers aren't that hard to get ahold of, and rose petals are easy as well. you don't want to use rose essential oils since it'll take too much, and the right grade of rose essential oil, which is pure essential oil or therapeutic, can be far too expensive to waste in a bath. Therefore, using the flower is usually best, but both of these flowers are relaxing.

Ingredients:

1. ½ Cup Rose Petals, Dried or Fresh
2. ¼ Cup Lavender Flowers, Dried or Fresh

*Directions:*

1. Mix your flowers together, adding them to a hot bath, and enjoy the relaxation it brings as your troubles melt away, including your stress. Make sure to soak for twenty to thirty minutes.

# Chapter 6. Essential Oils for Anxiety & Stress

Essential oils are great for stress and anxiety, and they're extremely easy to use. Stress is linked to a lot of illnesses, and it'll help to make sure it's under control. Essential are a great, healthy way to deal with your stress. They are both calming and stimulating, and they'll help to calm you while you work through your stress or just take a break from it.

You may find a restorative or calming effect from essential oils, usually depending on what you need. They work differently for different people, and sometimes they work differently at different times based on the individual's needs.

It'll help you to restore your balance, and it'll keep you from being fearful, angry, anxious, stressed or agitated. Remember that a top note is blended from five to twenty percent, a middle note is blended at fifty to eighty percent, and a base note is blended at five to twenty percent for the best results. This will tell you how much of each oil to use to get the right blend for you and your stress related issues.

**Essential Oil #1 Lavender**

Lavender is an extremely common essential oil to use for many things, especially for stress and anxiety. It's commonly referred to as a universal essential oil, and it helps with stress because it affects your body by calming it and the aroma is meant to sooth you. Diffusing lavender helps to bring about a much more peaceful environment that can bring you a sense of inner peace. Lavender is a middle note.

## Essential Oil #2 Cedarwood

Cedarwood is great due to its calming properties, and it isn't just great for stress and anxiety. It's also known to help people with ADHD and ADD. It's known to have a woody and warm scent, but it's still soft. It blends great with rosemary, clary sage, or cypress, and it stimulates the limbic region of your brain. The limbic region of your brain is the centre of your emotions, and it also stimulates the pineal gland. This helps to release melatonin, which will play an important role in making sure you're on and staying on the right sleep cycle. You can apply it directly to the stem of the brain, which is where the neck joins to the head. Of course, you may need to use a carrier oil. However, diffusing it works as well. It's a base note.

## Essential Oil #3 Jasmine

Jasmine is a stimulating aroma, and it'll help to uplift your spirits, which is great at producing more optimism and confidence. It's great if you're fighting with depression because of your stress, and it will help to relieve insomnia, headaches and promote relaxation. It can be applied topically, but it works just as well if you diffuse it into a room. It's meant to be a mood enhancer, and it's great if you blend it with lemongrass, mandarin, spearmint, rose, or even Melissa. It has a powerful scent, and it's extremely floral. However, remember that you need pure jasmine oil, and not synthetic jasmine oil, since it won't have the same properties. Jasmine oil can be expensive when pure, so it's not a common essential oil to use despite its usefulness, but it is recommended. Jasmine essential oil is also a base note.

**Essential Oil #4 Orange**

Orange essential oil, unlike jasmine, is actually easy to get ahold of, so it's more likely to be used on a day to day basis. It ca help with depression, and it boosts the immune systems as well. It can be diffused or even taken internally if you have an edible citrus oil. It's an enhancer, and is best when paired with lavender, rosewood, or cinnamon bark. It's a fresh and fruity scent, that's also sweet. However, don't apply it topically to uncovered skin and go in the sun for twelve hours afterwards. Use a carrier oil, or avoid direct sunlight. It could increase your risk of burning. Orange essential oil is considered to be a top note.

### Essential Oil #5 Rose

Rose essential oil is great, and it's known to be overpowering. You need a therapeutic grade oil, but it can be overpowering, so make sure to only apply a little and use a carrier oil when possible. It's an oil that's commonly used in a blend rather than on its own, but it promotes a sense of well-being, and it has a high frequency that will help to stimulate your mind and actually help to make sure that you're finding balance again. It blends well with different citrus oils, pine, patchouli, or even clary sage. It's spicy and floral. It's considered deep and sensual, but it's not to be used during pregnancy. Of course, be careful and look out for any cheap imitations, as they won't have the same effects, just like with jasmine oil. Rose is actually a middle to base note.

**Essential Oil #6 Valerian**

This essential oil is known to help with both stress and sleep, and it's great if you're diffusing it through the room. However, despite its use for sleep enhancement, for some people it can act as a mild stimulant. It doesn't have a pleasant aroma, or at least most people don't think so, which is why it's commonly used in blends. However, it has amazing effects on reducing both stress and anxiety. It can be applied topically as well, which is usually to the soles of your feet or even to your wrists. You can take it internally with a food grade essential oil in a supplement, or you can dilute a food grade into teaspoon of honey and then take it on its own or in a four once beverage. Never give it to children, especially children under six years old. Since it's not commonly diffused because of the smell, it's not recommended to use in a blend. Applying it topically is usually the preferred method.

## Essential Oil #7 Marjoram

Marjoram is known to be an herb of happiness, and a joy of the mountain, and it was used by both the Greeks and the Romans it works as a muscle relaxant, and it promotes sleep. It's great for migraine headaches, and commonly it is diffused for the best results. It pairs great with orange, lavender, chamomile, cedarwood, rosemary, or even nutmeg. It's considered to be a mild note that is spicy and green. However, it should always be avoided when you're pregnant. It's an equalizer and an enhancer. Marjoram is a middle note.

**Essential Oil #8 Orange Blossom**

Orange blossom is different than orange essential oil. It is relaxing, promotes confidence, hopefulness, sensuality, peace, and it's extremely calming. It is a middle note, and is sweet with a slightly bitter odor. It blends great with jasmine, lavender, and rose. It is a great way to boost your mood, and it's not at hard to get ahold of as other essential oils.

Orange blossom is commonly used as a blend and not by itself if you're looking for the best results.

**Essential Oil #9 Sandalwood**

It affects the brain's limbic system, helping to balance your immune system as well as your emotions. It can be applied both topically or diffused. Many people prefer to use a carrier oil when applying topically, and it is a modifier. It can blend with cypress, lemon, spruce, lemon, and patchouli. It is a base note, and it has a slightly minty and fruity scent. You need to use it with caution if you're pregnant, and many doctors will recommend that you do not use it at all. True sandalwood oil can be expensive because the supply of sandalwood trees is diminishing, so you need to be cautious about the quality of oil that you're getting, and it may be rather expensive.

## Essential Oil #10 Roman Chamomile

Roman chamomile is able to help with your sleep issues, and it can relax you, dispel anger, release old emotions, and reduce any anxiety and stress that you're feeling. It's best when applied topically, but you can diffuse it for results as well. If you're applying it topically, then take two drops, rubbing it on the temples, or even on the back of your neck. Since it promotes sleep, it's recommended to do so before going to bed, but you can also do so before you face a situation that is difficult for you. It can help you to express your feelings, and many people will actually apply it to their throat area for this result, commonly during meditation. It's great if you blend it with clary sage, rose, lavender or even geranium. It's a middle note, and it has a fresh and sweet scent. However, if you have sensitive skin you'll need to dilute it because it can irritate skin easily.

## Essential Oil #11 German Chamomile

Always make sure you're aware of the type of chamomile you're getting before you buy the essential oil, as German chamomile is different than Roman chamomile. It can dispel anger, and it brings your emotions back into balance. However, it's best if you're diffusing or inhaling it. It goes well with lavender, marjoram, lemongrass, spruce, or sandalwood. It's a middle note, and it has a deep and rich scent. However, it can irate sensitive skin, and it is not recommended to be used while pregnant.

# Chapter 7. Natural Habits You Can Stack

Your daily habits are going to actually cause or reduce stress. You need to make the choices that will help to make sure that your stress is actually being reduced instead of being added to when you're trying to manage it naturally. It won't be enough if you're just trying to make sure that you drink a stress reducing tea once a day. Your habits mean more than what you put in your body sometimes, and a drink just won't cut it even if it helps.

**Habit #1 Exercise Daily**

It has been proven that your body is more able to handle stress correctly if your physical body has been active. This can keep the physical effects of stress at bay, and it can help to make sure that your mental state is more equipped to handling stress as well. It doesn't have to be anything too hard, but you need to exercise for thirty minutes to an hour a day.

Two thirty minute sessions are known to work best, and you'll find that it'll help to make sure that you're prepared for stress. It'll also help you to sleep and feel more accomplished. Daily exercise actually gives you energy after time, and it'll help to make sure that you're prepared for anything that comes your way. Exercise itself can be a great way to de-stress as well, since it gives you a proper outlet for frustrations or anger.

**Habit #2 Don't Leave Chores**

You may think that your chores are actually dragging you down and causing more stress, but if you leave them, then you're going to worry about them, consciously or not. It's best to just get it out of the way, and that'll help to make sure that nothing is left for the next day. this is why making a chore list is usually best because even if you can't get all of your chores done in one day, then it'll help to make sure that you a plan. Having a plan will help to make sure that you don't feel overwhelmed, which often leads to stress.

Feeling like you have more chores than you have time, will cause you issues, and you need to manage it. For example, you need to stop leaving dirty dishes in the sink overnight. You're going to wake up to dirty dishes, knowing that you have even more of them because you didn't do them all in one day. So try to make time for a chore like that every day, but you may only need to vacuum the entire house every other day or every three days, depending on how messy your house tends to get on a regular basis. So you won't need it on your list every day.

## Habit #3 Compliment Yourselves

This is often hard to do. When you feel too stressed, you're going to feel insecure and depressed. Of course, this means it's extremely hard to make sure that you're doing what you need to avoid the stress and the depression. You need to find something that you can compliment yourself on. You can do it throughout the day, but try to do it at least once daily. In the morning is one of the easiest ways to compliment yourself because you're usually getting dressed in the morning.

Many people who are stressed won't actually feel like they look beautiful because they lack the confidence to do so. Tell yourself that your hair looks good, that you look smart, that you look ready to face the day, that your eyes are bright that day, or that you choose the right choice in clothes because they're flattering. Any compliment will help, and it'll boost your confidence, relieving some of the stress that you're feeling that day or stave off stress for at least a little while.

## Habit #4 Sleep on a Schedule

Stress is known to wreck your sleep, and not sleeping will actually cause more stress. It's a bad cycle, and it's one that you have to break if you want to decrease the amount of stress in your life. Stress can prevent you from actually sleeping the quantity you need to be, and it can actually stop you from getting the quality that you need as well.

You need to log in adequate hours if you want to enjoy the day ahead of you. It's important that you get eight to nine hours. This is why herbal teas or baths are great before bed, and it'll help to make sure that you're getting the sleep you need. Sometimes, you may even want to take something to naturally promote sleep if it gets too bad.

So start by getting on the proper schedule. Make sure you go to bed around the same time each night and get up around the same time. Often, you'll want to go to bed thirty minutes earlier and then get up thirty minutes earlier. It can help you to make sure that you're getting the right amount of sleep, and you can always take a nap later if you've still had a rough night. It'll help to make sure that you're not oversleeping, but you're getting the right amount of hours for you.

**Habit #5 Start Saying No**

Sometimes you have to say no. It may not seem like you're being selfish, but sometimes you need to say no to people. Sometimes you need to take that time for yourself, and you shouldn't be stuck doing things you don't have to for someone else if you don't want to. So just say no. learning to say no is usually hard, but it'll make you a happier person.

The people you keep around you should be there for you and not for what you can do for them. Real friends and good family will stay with you even if you can't do things for them. Occasionally it's find to do something for someone else just to help them out, even if it's a small inconvenience, but you'll often want to take that time and reserve it for yourself if you want to keep stress at bay.

## Habit #6 Schedule a Time to Stress

You do eventually have to deal with your stress, but most stressors don't have to be dealt with immediately. You'll find that commonly all you have to do is deal with it later. This should be a time when you're not busy and you have a clear mind. It can be after you do something else to help you with your stress to make sure your mind is clear, such as making sure that you've went for a jog, listened to music, meditated or even just had an herbal tea beforehand. If you have a time to worry about your stressors, then you won't feel the need to do so all the time, and you'll be able to successfully solve your problems by having the time and the right mindset.

**Stack Your Habits:**

Never just use one habit. You should always stack your habits. The more you stack, the less stress you'll feel. If you're making the right choices in your life, then you're going to be less stressed. You're going to be able to recognize that your life is going well, and you'll be able to feel healthier and be healthier, mentally, emotionally and physically because of your habits and the stress reduction that follows.

# Chapter 8. Stress Relieving Face Masks

Stress has an effect on your physical body, and sometimes that means it can cause you to have acne and blackheads. Of course, this is where you're going to want to enjoy a facemask. It'll help to clear up your skin once again, but it'll also help to make sure that you have everything you need to distress. Sometimes, it's as simple as taking the time out of your day to take care of yourself, like you would with a facemask that will help with your stress. Of course, there are many scents and sensations that can help you to feel less stressed as well, and many people are surprised at how feeling beautiful and confident can contribute to stress relief as well.

**Face Mask #1 A Papaya Mask**

It can help to reduce wrinkles, and it'll even help to make sure that you're enjoying the feeling of clean, healthy skin. Make sure to rinse it off with warm water, and it'll bring the scent of the tropics to you, which often helps you to center yourself. You can actually practice breathing exercises while enjoying this facemask.

Ingredients:

1. 3 Tablespoons Papaya, Blended & Mashed
2. 1/3 Cup Oatmeal
3. 1 Tablespoon Honey, Raw

*Directions:*

1. Mix all ingredients and apply smoothly to your face. Let sit for five to ten minutes.

2. It should dry and harden before you remove it. Wash off with warm water, and gently pat the area dry.

**Facemask #2 Rose Facemask**

Everyone believes roses are a relaxing scent, and it's actually been proven to be relaxing to the body. Many people will release tension, and rose oil is great if you're looking for something to tone your face and make sure that it's rejuvenated at the same time as you're letting the stress melt away.

Ingredients:

1. 1/3 Cup Oatmeal
2. 1 Tablespoon Honey, Raw
3. 1 Teaspoon Rose Infused Oil

*Directions:*

1. Mix everything together, and then apply it to your face.
2. Let dry. You should let it sit for ten to twelve minutes before washing with cool water, patting the area dry.

## Facemask #3 Lavender & Honey Facemask

Honey is great for your skin, and it'll help to erase the look of stress right from your face. It gives you a youthful look and makes sure that your body is relaxing to the scent of lavender. From lavender flowers to lavender oil, this is a facemask that helps to make sure you have it all. Of course, fresh lavender flowers are needed, but some people believe dried flowers will work most of the time.

Ingredients:

1. ½ Cup Lavender Flowers, Bruised

2. ¼ Cup Honey, Raw
3. ¼ Cup Oatmeal
4. 3-5 Drops Lavender Essential Oil

*Directions:*

1. Mix everything together in a medium bowl, and apply it to your face.
2. Let sit for ten to twelve minutes, and wash off with cool or warm water, patting the area dry afterwards.

**Facemask #4 Chamomile Face Mask**

Chamomile tea is great for your skin, and it can be a great way to sooth away wrinkles and acne. With honey, it helps as well, and that's all you need except for maybe a little more oats to help get your skin and your stress back on track. It's not just the taste of chamomile that relaxes you, but the smell as well, and that's one of the reasons chamomile tea is usually best drunk hot. However, it works great in this facemask remedy.

Ingredients:

1. 1/3 Cup Oats
2. ¼ Cup Honey, Raw
3. ½ Cup Chamomile Tea

*Directions:*

1. You will want your chamomile tea to be prepared in advance, and you can make a full cup or a half a cup, but you're going to only want to use half for this facemask recipe or it'll come out far too watery.
2. Take a small bowl, and mix all of your ingredients together, applying it to your face, and let it sit for eight to ten minutes.

3. Wash off with cool or warm water, letting it dry or patting your face dry gently.

**Facemask #5 Jasmine Facemask**

If you have jasmine flowers growing in your backyard, then you're in luck. Jasmine is actually a relaxing scent, and the crushed flowers have been known to inspire thought, relax your body, and keep stress at bay. The crushed flowers are usually best, but you can make it with just essential oil if necessary.

Ingredients:

1. ½ Cup Jasmine Flowers, Crushed
2. 5-6 Drops Jasmine Essential Oil
3. ¼ Cup Honey, Raw
4. ¼ Cup Oats, Raw

*Direction:*

1. Mix everything together in a small to medium bowl, making sure that the jasmine flowers are crushed and bruised. If you do not have jasmine flowers, then you can increase the oats to a half cup and increase the drops to eight or ten.
2. Apply to the face, and let dry for eight to twelve minutes, removing with cool water, and patting the area dry.

**Facemask #6 Vanilla Paste Facemask**

Vanilla is also known to be a relaxing scent, and you can make a paste out of the extract or essential oil, which is actually extremely easy to find. You can also add a dash of cinnamon in there to give it an exotic smell and keep acne at bay. You can release tension with this wonderful facemask, and it's edible too.

Ingredients:

1. 2 Teaspoons Vanilla Extract
2. 1/8 Cup Honey, Raw
3. 2 Large Bananas, Mashed
4. 1 Teaspoon Cinnamon

*Directions:*

1. Take everything and mix it thoroughly together in a bowl, and then apply it to your face. Let sit for six to eight minutes. You can leave it on longer if desired.
2. Wash off with cool water, patting the area dry.

## Facemask #7 Cinnamon & Oats

Cinnamon is known to sharpen your mind and bring a sense of wellbeing. Add some sweet almond oil, which is great for your skin and makes you look youthful and clears up acne, and you have a wonderful facemask.

Ingredients:

1. ¼ Cup Sweet Almond Oil
2. 3 Teaspoons Cinnamon
3. 1/8 Cup Oats, Raw

*Direction:*

1. Mix together, and add more cinnamon and oats if necessary.
2. Apply to the face, and let sit for eight to ten minutes. Wash off gently with warm or cool water, patting the area dry.

**Remember:**

A facemask is great, but only if you're in the mood for it. You have to try to want to relax before you do, and you need to set time aside for it. It's not going to help you if you put on a facemask and then try to do the chores while it dries. It'll still help your skin, but it's unlikely to help your stress nearly as much as it could have. Put time aside for it during the day, usually during the evening is best, and you'll see much better results. Try to relax when you're using a facemask, and start with breathing exercises if possible. Make sure to breathe through your nose, since the scents are what's relaxing you as well as the feeling of exfoliating your skin. So, half the battle is being able to smell the facemask.

# Chapter 9. Extra Tips & Tricks to Help

Of course, there are some extra tips and tricks that you can use to help you with your stress as well. There's absolutely no need to carry around a large amount of stress in your life. It will naturally happen, but it doesn't have to build up.

**Bonus Tip #1 Prepare for the Day**

Sometimes it's best to actually prepare for the next day if you don't want to be stressed. You still need to be flexible, but you'll find that there are many ways you can still prepare for the day to make it go a little smoother. If your day is going smoother, then you're much likely to actually be able to handle stressful situations or even dismiss stressful situations entirely.

One way to prepare for the day is to make sure that your clothes are laid out and prepared. If your morning routine goes smoothly, then you're much more likely to have a smooth day overall. You will also want to outline anything you need to get done the next day, but don't add anything that isn't important. You don't want to plan out every moment, but important events should be taken care of.

**Bonus Tip #2 Focus on One Thing**

Sometimes you can't focus on a large amount of things. Sometimes, you just need to focus on what you're doing right then and there. Otherwise, even things that shouldn't be that stressful could be far too overwhelming, making the stress seem unmanageable. If you make sure that you're concentrating on the task at hand, then you'll be able to better perform that task.

You'll be able to accomplish that job, and then move on. When you move on, then you'll be able to mark something off your list, or it'll help you to enjoy the moment if you're doing something relaxing. This is where your plan comes in handy because you'll be able to live in the moment, focusing on what's at hand, while still making sure that you don't forget anything important.

**Bonus Tip #3 Be Silly Sometimes**

It isn't something that you can do all the time, but sometimes you can't always be serious. You'll need to make sure that you have time to indulge your inner child. Allow yourself to be silly. It doesn't have to be in front of anyone if you're self-conscious, but it should be done at least once a day. It can be okay to be immature, and it's a great break from living the stressful life of an adult. It may only be for a moment or for an hour, but doing something silly will help to banish a good majority of your stress away.

**Bonus Tip #4 Chew Gum**

This may seem silly, but chewing gum is known to help relieve stress. It doesn't matter what gum you chew, but mint is known to be a relief as well, which will usually help too. Chewing gum can reduce cortisol levels, and this is a great way to help alleviate your stress immediately. It won't actually solve any of your problems, but it'll allow you to look at your problems a little more calmly so that you can solve them yourself. So having gum on hand is always a good idea.

## Bonus Tip #5 Have Sex

If possible, have sex. Sex is known to help reduce your stress, and it's extremely helpful if you have someone you love to have sex with. It can make a healthy relationship, and it can ensure that your stress is lessened almost instantly. It can increase physical symptoms of stress, and it relieves the tension in your body, reduce headaches, and keep your hormones in balance.

## Bonus Tip #6 Take a Nap

Sleep is important to your health, and it's important to your stress as well, as stated before. If you are more rested, then you are more likely to handle stressful situations and embrace the day ahead of you. If you're tired, then you shouldn't just ignore it. You may want to take a nap, and if you need to you can set an alarm, but it's not always necessary. Napping will also reduce your cortisol levels, relieving stress and the physical symptoms that come with stress.

**Always Face It**

Just remember that no matter how much you reduce your stress, you need to face it as well. You can't just hide from all of your issues. You have to cope with them and then deal with them. Cut what's stressful out of your life, including negative influences. You don't need negative influences in your life, and you need to remember that sometimes you need to just cut them out. You can't fix everything, but you need to at least fix what you can. Deal with what you can, and cope with everything else. Sometimes coping mechanisms are just meant to help to make sure that you are in a more reasonable state of mind that will help you to completely solve your stressful problems.

www.ingramcontent.com/pod-product-compliance
Lightning Source LLC
Chambersburg PA
CBHW052203110526
44591CB00012B/2058